FATTY LIVER DISEASE DIET

A Beginner's Step-by-Step Guide with Recipes and a Meal Plan

Copyright © 2020 Bruce Ackerberg
All rights reserved. No portion of this book may be reproduced in any form without permission from the publisher, except as permitted by U.S. copyright law.

TABLE OF CONTENTS

Introduction
Chapter 1 – What is Fatty liver?
Chapter 2 – Fatty liver Diet
Chapter 3 – Steps In Maintaining A Fatty liver Diet
Chapter 4 - Diet Plan And Sample Recipes for Fatty liver Patients
Chapter 5 – Lifestyle Changes
Conclusion

Disclaimer
By reading this disclaimer, you are accepting the terms of the disclaimer in full. If you disagree with this disclaimer, please do not read the guide. The content in this guide is provided for informational and educational purposes only.

This guide is not intended to be a substitute for the original work of this diet plan. At most, this guide is intended to be a beginner's supplement to the original work for this diet plan and never act as a direct substitute. This guide is an overview, review, and commentary on the facts of that diet plan.

All product names, diet plans, or names used in this guide are for identification purposes only and are the property of their respective owners. The use of these names does not imply endorsement. All other trademarks cited herein are the property of their respective owners.

None of the information in this guide should be accepted as independent medical or other professional advice.

The information in the guide has been compiled from various sources that are deemed reliable. It has been analyzed and summarized to the best of the Author's ability, knowledge, and belief. However, the Author cannot guarantee the accuracy and thus should not be held liable for any errors.

You acknowledge and agree that the Author of this guide will not be held liable for any damages, costs, expenses, resulting from the application of the information in this guide, whether directly or indirectly. You acknowledge and agree that you assume all risk and responsibility for any action you undertake in response to the information in this guide.

You acknowledge and agree that by continuing to read this guide, you will (where applicable, appropriate, or necessary) consult a qualified medical professional on this information. The information in this guide is not intended to be any sort of medical advice and should not be used in lieu of any medical advice by a licensed and qualified medical professional.

Always seek the advice of your physician or another qualified health provider with any issues or questions you might have regarding any sort of medical condition. Do not ever disregard any qualified professional medical advice or delay seeking that advice because of anything you have read in this guide.

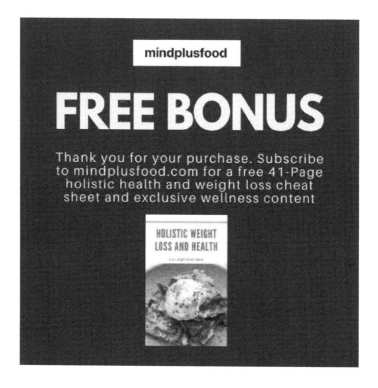

INTRODUCTION

Fatty liver is a condition that currently affects almost a third of the US population. This is mainly due to excessive alcohol consumption, unhealthy food choices, and sedentary lifestyles. Left unchecked, fatty liver can cause damage to the liver and lead to serious medical conditions such as liver fibrosis or scarring, and cirrhosis, which can be fatal.

As of this writing, there are no FDA approved medications for the direct treatment of fatty liver. Fortunately, and if diagnosed early, this condition is easily reversible by making changes in the patient's diet and lifestyle.

That's where this guide can help. It's written for people who were diagnosed with fatty liver and are hoping to eat healthier.

The guide starts with important information on the disease and the symptoms that accompany it. A chapter is devoted to listing the foods shown to help with the treatment and reversal of fatty liver according to studies. A diet and lifestyle change plan is also included in the book to help the patient in the journey to living healthier.

CHAPTER 1 – WHAT IS FATTY LIVER?

Also known as hepatic steatosis, fatty liver happens when there is a buildup of fat in the liver. Although it is normal to have a small amount of fat in the liver, too much of it can cause a serious health problem.

The liver is the human body's second-largest organ. Its basic function is to assist in the processing and storing of nutrients from food and drinks and also filtering out harmful substances from the blood. In addition, the liver is also responsible for the metabolism of medicines, important clotting factors, and the production of glucose.

Too much fat in the liver can cause it to become inflamed. This can damage the liver and eventually cause irreversible damage or scarring and in severe cases, death since as some sources claim, the liver is the greatest immune defense of the body; once it fails, all else follows.

If a person who drinks too much alcohol develops fatty liver, the condition is called alcoholic fatty liver or AFLD.
If a person who doesn't drink alcohol is diagnosed with the disease, it's called non-alcoholic fatty liver or NAFLD.
Currently, 25 to 30% of people in Europe and the United States are suffering from NAFLD according to a report released by researchers from the World Journal of Gastroenterology.

What are the Symptoms?
In most cases, fatty liver is asymptomatic which means there are

no noticeable symptoms--- which may be deemed as usual symptoms of normal illnesses.

To be more specific, alcoholic fatty liver may also cause:
- Nausea
- Fever
- Jaundice; and
- Vomiting

While below are some symptoms which may be experienced by people with nonalcoholic fatty liver:
- Unexplained weight loss
- Jaundice
- Decreased appetite
- Swollen legs
- Itchy skin

In general, patients may initially experience general exhaustion or feel pain and discomfort in the upper right side of the abdomen.

When fatty liver is left unchecked, a person suffering from it can develop complications, one of which is liver scarring. This condition is called fibrosis (stage 2 liver disease) and if it gets worse, it can lead to liver cirrhosis (stage 3 liver disease), a potentially deadly medical condition.

Some symptoms of liver cirrhosis include:
- Significant weight loss
- Loss of appetite
- Fatigue
- Weakness
- Itchy skin
- Yellow eyes and skin
- Nosebleeds
- Abdominal pain and swelling
- Swelling legs
- Confusion

- Enlargement of the breast in men

What Causes Fatty Liver?
Fatty liver occurs when the body is producing too much fat and it isn't being metabolized efficiently or fast enough. The excess fat is then stored in the liver where it can accumulate and cause the disease.

There are a variety of factors that can cause this fat build-up. As previously mentioned, drinking too much alcohol can cause AFLD, which is usually the initial stage of liver diseases that are associated with alcohol consumption.
But for people who drink alcohol in moderation or those that totally abstain from it and still develop NAFLD, the cause is less clear.

One or a few of these factors are considered to be potential causes:
- High blood sugar or diabetes
- Obesity
- Resistance to insulin
- High-fat levels in the blood, especially triglycerides

The following can also cause NAFLD but they're less common:
- Rapid weight loss
- Pregnancy
- Infections like hepatitis C
- Side effects due to certain medications which include tamoxifen, methotrexate, valproic acid, and amiodarone.
- Exposure to some toxins

Certain human genes have also been found to increase the risks of having NAFLD.

How is Fatty Liver Diagnosed?
Diagnosis of fatty liver include gathering the patient's medical history, conducting a physical exam, and doing one or more of the following tests:
- Blood test for elevated liver enzymes
- Imaging tests such MRI, CT scan, and ultrasound

- Liver biopsy

Fatty liver Treatment

There are currently no approved medications for the treatment of fatty liver. But, in more severe cases of fatty liver wherein patients already have compromised airways, brain damage, and impaired swallowing reflexes, dietary intervention/ management through oral or tube feeding is made under the supervision of a dietitian and a doctor. The diet consists of complex carbohydrates, fats, and proteins in liquid form to give proper nutrition to the patient.

Fortunately, fatty liver is reversible in many cases and is easily accomplished by lifestyle changes like losing excess weight, avoiding or limiting alcohol, and making changes to the patient's diet.

CHAPTER 2 – FATTY LIVER DIET

One of the most effective approaches to fatty liver is through losing excess body fat. Health experts agree that 70% of weight loss is due to diet.

Although there are no FDA approved drugs for the fatty liver yet, doctors agree that losing around 10% of the person's body weight is a good start, especially to patients who are obese.

NAFLD has been found most common for patients who live a sedentary lifestyle and those who consume mainly highly-processed foods.

Basic Components Of The Fatty liver Diet
A diet plan for people who have fatty liver should include the following:

- Lots of vegetables and fruits
- High-fiber foods like whole grains and legumes
- Reduced consumption of salt, sugar, refined carbohydrates, trans fat, and saturated fat
- No alcohol

Basically, the patient should undergo a reduced-calorie, low-fat diet to help in losing the excess weight.

Foods to Include in a Fatty liver Diet Plan

- **Greens**. In a study, broccoli has been found to be effective in helping prevent fat building in the livers of mice. Consuming more green vegetables like Brussels sprouts, spinach, and kale might also help with weight loss. There are a lot of vegetarian recipes that are full of flavor but low in calories.

- **Coffee**. Research has shown that those with fatty liver who also drink coffee are less susceptible to liver damage than those who don't. It's thought that the caffeine in this beverage reduces the levels of abnormal liver enzymes for those people that have high risks for liver diseases.

- **Fish**. Especially the fatty ones such as sardines, salmon, trout, and tuna, contain significant amounts of healthy omega-3 fatty acids. Omega-3 fatty acids have been found to help in improving fat levels in the liver and significantly reduce inflammation.

- **Tofu**. Soybeans have high protein content. Tofu is a soy product that has high protein content but a very low fat amount. A study made on rats by the University of Illinois showed that soy protein reduces liver fat buildup.

- **Walnuts**. These contain high amounts of omega-3 fatty acids which, as previously discussed, have shown to be beneficial in improving the liver function for patients diagnosed with fatty liver.

- **Oatmeal**. Carbohydrates consumed by patients with fatty liver should come from whole grains like oatmeal. Complex carbohydrates release a steady amount of energy and the fiber content satiates which is important in weight maintenance.

- **Low-fat dairy.** Whey protein might be able to help in protecting the liver from damage and this is important for those with fatty liver. Milk and other dairy products have high whey protein content but it's recommended those with reduced fat content.

- **Avocado**. It might be high in fat content but these are the healthy ones. Research suggests that healthy fats and certain chemicals found in avocado can slow down liver damage. Avocados are also fiber-rich which helps in weight control.

- **Olive oil**. It's one of the healthiest and more readily available oils in the market. Olive oil is rich in omega-3 fatty acids and is much healthier when used for food preparation compared to shortening, butter, or margarine. Research shows that it can lower the number of liver enzymes and also help control weight.

- **Sunflower seeds**. The vitamin E content of the nutty-tasting sunflower seeds can protect the liver from damage due to its anti-oxidant properties.

- **Green tea.** From aiding with sleep to lowering cholesterol, green tea has shown many medical and health benefits. Initial studies show that green tea helps by interfering with fat absorption. It might also help with improving liver function and reducing fat storage in the organ.

- **Garlic**. It doesn't just add a lot of flavor and aroma to food but garlic powder supplements are also showing potential in the reduction of excess body weight for people with fatty liver.

- **Healthy fats.** Fat is still needed even in people prone to fatty liver disease. Choosing healthy fats such as fish oil, nuts, vegetable oils, omega- 3 fatty acids is smarter since they are unsaturated and do not stay in the liver.

Foods to Avoid

The following foods should be avoided or the consumption limited for patients with fatty liver. These contribute to increased blood sugar levels and weight gain which should be avoided when treating the disease.

- Alcohol. It's not only the major cause for the disease but also for other organ diseases.
- Fried food. These are soaked in saturated fat and generally high in calories.
- Added sugar. Sugary foods such as cookies, candies, fruit juices, and soda should be avoided. High levels of sugar in the blood can increase liver fat buildup.
- Pasta, rice, and bread. Especially the white ones because the flour used has been highly processed. These can raise blood sugar levels. Opt for brown rice and whole wheat bread and pasta as these have higher fiber content that can help eliminate fat and unhealthy cholesterol from the body.
- Salt. Salt is linked to water retention and also causes fat buildup and high blood pressure but it's an essential ingredient of most foods. Limit consumption to no more than 1.5 grams per day.
- Red meat. Avoid deli meats and beef because these have high saturated fat content.

CHAPTER 3 – STEPS IN MAINTAINING A FATTY LIVER DIET

Treating fatty liver with food is basically eating healthy. Here are some tips to consider for people with this condition

Eating Regular Meals
Eating regularly makes controlling appetite easier because it can reduce cravings and helps in planning healthy meals. Aim to have 3 major meals per day.

Follow the Mediterranean Diet Pyramid
Fruits and vegetables, legumes, seeds, nuts, cereals, and whole-grain bread should take up most of the calories the patient consumes. Proteins should come from lean sources like fish, chicken breasts, and eggs. Low-fat dairy also provides additional protein, calcium, and other nutrients.
When the body gets enough nutrition coming from these food groups, craving for high sugar and high fat is greatly reduced.

Choose Healthier Drinks
Water is still the best beverage, especially for those people who are trying to lose weight. It contains zero calories and drinking a glass before a meal reduces food intake. Avoid drinks with too much sugar like juices, sports drinks, cordials, and sodas. Also, avoid alcohol as it can worsen fatty liver. Not only does it give more work for the liver, when alcohol calorie doesn't get burned,

but they are also stored as fat in other parts of the body as well.

Reduce Portion Sizes
Replace that dinner plate with a salad plate. Studies show that the bigger the plate, the more food is consumed. Use smaller bowls and plates to reduce calorie intake.

Choose Healthier Alternatives
Eat more vegetables, fruits, legumes, and wholegrain, high-fiber cereals and bread. These satiate faster and longer but with fewer calories. In cooking, you can opt to skip table salt or sugar and lean into using spices. These improve the meal flavors, and at the same time, have better effects on health.

Here are examples of replacing food choices with better alternatives:
- Instead of a 1/3 bowl of muesli, eat a 2/3 bowl of oats
- Instead of a glass of fruit drink, eat 3 pieces of fruits
- Instead of 40 grams of chocolate, eat 2 slices multigrain bread

Both choices have the same calorie content but the latter is more filling than the former.

Plan Ahead
Planning meals ahead can help limit instances of impulse eating, the temptation of grabbing a takeaway, and other spur-of-the-moment food choices. Prepare a meal plan for the whole week and shop for the ingredients in the supermarket. Cooking meals and storing them in the refrigerator or freezer also helps a lot in controlling calorie intake. In addition, avoid going to the groceries when hungry to avoid impulsive, unhealthy buys.

CHAPTER 4 - DIET PLAN AND SAMPLE RECIPES FOR FATTY LIVER PATIENTS

Sample Meal Plan

A typical meal plan for a patient with fatty liver might look like this:

Meal	Menu
Breakfast	- Hot oatmeal (8 Oz.), mixed with almond butter (2 tsp.) and sliced banana (1 pc.) - Coffee with skim or low-fat milk (1 cup)
Lunch	- Salad greens with olive oil and balsamic vinegar dressing - Grilled chicken, 3 oz. - Baked small potato - Cooked carrots or broccoli, 1 cup - Apple, 1 pc. - Milk, 1 glass
Snack	- Raw veggies with 2 tbsp. of hummus or sliced apples with 1 tbsp. peanut butter
Dinner	- Mixed-bean salad, small - Grilled salmon, 3 Oz. - Cooked broccoli, 1 cup

| | | - Whole-grain roll, 1 pc
- Mixed berries, 1 cup
- Milk, 1 glass |

Another sample meal plan for a whole day:

Meal	Menu
Breakfast	- High-fiber cereal with low-fat milk or multigrain bread (2 slices) with tomato / baked beans / peanut butter / mushrooms / cottage cheese - Fruit, 1 pc. - Water
Morning Tea	- Fruit (1 pc) / Greek yogurt (100 – 200 g) / oatmeal biscuits (2 pcs.) / fruit bread (1 thin slice) / grainy crackers with tomato and cottage cheese (2 pcs.) / raw nuts (5 to 6 pcs.)
Lunch	- 1 wrap / 1 bread roll / multigrain bread (2 slices) - Green salad with low fat cheese / chicken / salmon / tuna - Water
Afternoon Tea	- Fruit (1 pc) / Greek yogurt (100 – 200 g) / oatmeal biscuits (2 pcs.) / fruit bread (1 thin slice) / grainy crackers with tomato and cottage cheese (2 pcs.) / raw nuts (5 to 6 pcs.)
Dinner	- 120 g lean chicken / eggs / chicken / legumes - Vegetables (zucchini / spinach / peas / cauliflower / carrots / cabbage / broccoli / beans - Whole wheat pasta (1 cup) / Brown rice (2/3 cup) / sweet potato (1/2 cup) / medium potato (1 pc.) - Water

Just because you're going low-calorie does not mean you have to put up with bland food. There are ways to add flavor to any food without putting in too much salt or sugar. Here are some sample recipes that are low in calorie content but big in flavor.

Sample Recipes

Baked Salmon

Ingredients:
Lemons, 2 pcs, thinly sliced
Salmon fillet, (around 3 lbs.)
Kosher salt
Black pepper, freshly ground
Butter, melted, 6 tbsp.
Honey, 2 tbsp.
Garlic, minced, 3 cloves
Thyme leaves, chopped, 1 tsp.
Dried oregano, 1 tsp.
Fresh parsley, chopped, for garnish

Instructions:
1. Preheat the oven to 350 degrees. Use a foil to line a rimmed baking sheet. Grease it with cooking oil spray.
2. Lay the lemon slices on the center of the foil to form an even layer.
3. Season the salmon fillet on both sides with kosher salt and freshly ground black pepper.
4. Place fillet on top of the layer of lemon slices.
5. Whisk together oregano, thyme, garlic, honey, and butter in a small bowl. Pour this mixture over the salmon fillet and fold the foil up and around the salmon
6. Bake for 25 minutes or until the salmon is cooked through.
7. Garnish with chopped fresh parsley and serve hot.

Grilled Chicken Breast

Ingredients:
Skinless, boneless, chicken breasts, 4 pcs.
Sugar, 1 tbsp.
Garlic powder, 1 tsp.
Italian seasoning, 2 tbsp.
Pepper, 1 tbsp.
Salt, 1 tbsp.
Lemon juice, 2 tbsp.
Worcestershire sauce, 3 tbsp.
Dijon mustard, 2 tbsp.
Cider vinegar, ¼ cup
Olive oil, 1/3 cup

Instructions:
1. Combine all of the ingredients in Ziploc bag or large bowl. Massage or toss until well combined.
2. Marinade the chicken breasts for at least 30 minutes. You can also refrigerate for up to 4 hours.
3. Preheat the grill to medium to medium-high heat.
4. Place marinated chicken breasts on the grill and cook for 7 to 8 minutes. Flip them over and cook for another 7 to 8 minutes.
5. Take the chicken off the grill and place in a serving plate. Let them rest for 3 to 5 minutes

Mixed Bean Salad

Ingredients:
Canned mixed bean salad
Spring onions, 2 stalks, finely chopped
Celery, 2 sticks, thinly sliced
Tomato, large, 1 pc, deseeded then finely diced
Salt
Freshly ground black pepper
Dressing:
Olive oil, 3 tbsp
White wine vinegar, 1 tbsp
Sugar, 1 tsp
Dijon mustard, 2 tsp
Fresh tarragon, chopped, 1 tbsp
Fresh parsley, chopped, 1 tbsp

Instructions:
1. Put mixed beans, spring onions, celery, and tomato in a salad bowl. Add salt and pepper to taste. Mix well.
2. In a separate bowl, mix the ingredients for the dressing until well combined.
3. Pour the dressing on the salad and toss well together.

Smoothie for Liver Detox

Ingredients:
Fresh turmeric, 1 inch
Shredded raw beets, ½ cup
Raw spinach leaves, 1 cup

Fresh apple, ½ piece or Unsweetened apple sauce, ½ cup
Unsweetened almond milk, coconut water, or choice milk, 1 cup
Lemon juice from ½ or 1 whole lemon

Instructions
1. Chop roughly the apple and turmeric.
2. Shred the beets using a cheese grater.
3. Put all the ingredients in a blender.
4. Blend high until they are completely smooth.

Oatmeal Almond Cookies

Ingredients:
Almond flour, ¾ cup
Cinnamon, ½ tsp
Cranberries, dried and chopped into smaller bits
Gluten-free rolled oats, ¾ cup
Maple syrup, ¼ cup
Salt, a pinch
Optional: Cacao nibs, 2 tbsp

Instructions:
1. Preheat your oven to 350 degrees Fahrenheit.
2. Put the oats in the food processor, blender, or spice grinder and pulse until the oats are already ground into a meal. Put the ground oats in a bowl. Add the cinnamon, almond flour, and salt. Mix the ingredients well.
3. Pour the coconut oil into the bowl. Smash lightly into the flour using the back of a spoon. Put in the maple syrup, and mix it well.
4. Stir the cranberries and cacao nibs in.
5. Line the prepared baking sheet with Silpat or parchment paper. To scoop the cookies on the baking sheet, use a ¼ measuring cup and flatten the cookies until they are almost half-inch thick.
6. Bake the cookies for fifteen minutes.

How to get used to the Fatty Liver Diet
It may be easy to read, think, and try changing your lifestyle in order to be healthy. But, it is a given fact that changing one's lifestyle is not easy to do and maintain. So, the following are tips on how to maintain the diet and achieve your goal of a healthier liver.

Take it slowly. Every process is composed of a series of steps. And these steps should be taken seriously as this will lead you to the next. Thus, doing this diet is not an overnight thing. You can first start making healthier choices. Then, follow it up with regular exercise if you have already adapted to doing a healthier diet. Do not worry about doing it all together as this will only stress you and may prevent you from continuing to do so.

Trust the process. As mentioned in the previous tip, dieting is not an overnight thing. So, do not expect to see changes immediately. The fat in your liver took time to build up, thus it will also require time, discipline, and consistency in order to go back to normal. Just follow what is suggested and stick to it.

Be consistent. Losing weight is a step in having a healthier liver. But it doesn't mean that you lose weight, you also lose the fat in your liver. So, be happy when there are positive changes that are happening in your body. It means that you are already doing a great job. But what makes the job you are doing even better is if you continue to do what you have started.

Choose foods and activities that are comfortable for you. Even though there are suggested food items in this book, it doesn't mean that your options are limited to those. You can ask your doctor, dietitian, or do your research on similar food items that provide the same function and nutrient content. If you do not like almonds, you can opt for hazelnuts. If you do not like beets, you may try carrots. As long as it offers the same function, do as you please. Nothing's more discouraging if you are forced to eat what you don't like. It's the same with activities. If you are more comfortable working out in your home, then you can opt to do cardio exercises or aerobics in place instead of running, cycling, or running which requires you to go to places. It's your diet, so it's your choice.

Think about the long-term benefits. Are you afraid of the consequences which may be brought by fatty liver disease? Take this as a motivation to start or continue this diet. Would you rather pay thousands of bucks (or more) for expensive maintenance, regular hospital visits, and the worst-case--- hospitalization? Or would you rather eat healthier, exercise regularly, and avoid food that may affect your liver? You choose.

CHAPTER 5 – LIFESTYLE CHANGES

Treating fatty liver disease and reversing the damage is all about lowering body weight. A 10 percent reduction in excess weight is enough to improve enzyme levels in the liver according to doctors.

Aside from the diet, another recommendation from doctors is for those with fatty liver to make a change in their lifestyles. Most patients diagnosed with NAFLD live a sedentary life with very little to no physical activity.

Here are some changes the patient should make to improve liver health.

Avoid Alcohol
This can't be reiterated enough. The liver goes through a lot of stress during alcohol consumption since it is the one breaking down alcohol calories, not the stomach. Imagine that stress on an already diseased liver.

Lose Weight
But not rapidly. Losing 1 to 2 pounds per week should be the goal. And this may be done by deducting 500 kilocalories from your daily food intake. That means setting aside two muffins, one large fries, or almost a quarter pounder and a bottle of soda every day. Shedding off those extra pounds lower inflammation and prevents further injury to the liver.

Exercise
Aerobic has shown to be most effective in cutting fat levels in the

liver. Walk, jog, or run regularly. Physical exercise also lowers inflammation. Exercise at least 3 times a week.

Manage Diabetes

For patients who are also suffering from diabetes, they should consult their doctor for proper management. The inability of the body to process sugar properly due to diabetes puts additional stress to the liver.

Lower Cholesterol Levels

Keep triglycerides and cholesterol levels down. This can be done through medication or eating a plant-based diet, and regular exercise. In addition, fiber-rich foods such as beans, oatmeal, nuts, fruits, and vegetables, help in reducing the bad cholesterol levels.

Benefits of the Fatty Liver Diet Plan

No more nasty symptoms. Although the fatty liver disease may show little to no distinctive symptoms. Most symptoms such as confusion, fatigue, fever, abdominal pain, loss of appetite, and physical weakness are a hassle for your everyday life. So, doing the diet may help alleviate these symptoms since the diet mostly consists of healthier food options.

Less risk for other diseases. Experts say that fatty liver disease is associated with several diseases such as diabetes, obesity, protein-energy malnutrition, hypertension, and hyper cholesterol. Since the diet not only involves the consumption of healthy foods but also recommendations to do regular exercise, the risk to the mentioned diseases may also be lessened. It's like hitting a ton of birds with one stone.

Worry-free life. Once you have to get rid of the fatty liver, you have already lessened your risk for lifestyle diseases that may induce other complications. Thus, doing this diet will make you get rid of the unfavorable fatty liver disease symptoms and the difficulty in doing normal daily physical activities. It also strengthens your immune system because the diet is high in vitamins and minerals that help keep the body and its organs functioning well.

BONUS RECIPES

Green Smoothie

Ingredients

- 6 dandelion greens, chopped (about 1 cup)
- 4 kale leaves, stems removed and chopped (about 2 ½ cups)
- 1 Meyer or organic lemon, peeled and sliced into 1" chunks
- 1 small banana (optional) peeled and broken into 1" pieces
- 1 fuji apple, cut into 1" chunks
- 1 teaspoon grated ginger (optional)
- 2 cups Filtered water

Instructions

Place all ingredients, along with 2 cups water, into blender

Blend on high speed for 1-2 minutes until very smooth.

Add more water as necessary.

Turkey sandwich

Ingredients

- 2 oz whole wheat pita bread
- 3 oz roasted turkey, sliced
- 2 slices tomato
- A few leaves of romaine lettuce
- 1 tsp mustard
- ½ C grapes

Detox Juice

Ingredients
1 beet, scrubbed
one handful of greens, washed
1 apple
1 cucumber, peeled
1 lemon, peeled

Instructions:

Juice all ingredients and stir

Lentil Soup

Ingredients:

1 tbsp vegetable oil
1 cup diced onion ½ cup
diced carrot ½ cup
diced celery 4 cups vegetable or chicken broth 1 cup
dried red lentils well rinsed ¼ tsp
dried thyme
Salt and freshly ground pepper ½ cup
chopped fresh flat-leaf parsley (a sprinkle)

Instructions:
In a large saucepan, heat oil over medium heat.
Sauté onion, carrot and celery until they are soft.
This can be 5 minutes. Add broth, lentils and thyme.
Then bring to a boil.
Reduce heat, cover and simmer for 20 minutes or until lentils are soft.
Remove from heat.
Transfer soup into a blender.
Purée on high speed until creamy
Season with salt and pepper
Ladle into bowls and garnish with parsley

Ragi Oat Crackers with a Cucumber Dip

For the ragi and oat crackers

1. Combine all the ingredients in a deep bowl and knead into a stiff dough using enough water.
2. Divide the dough into 2 equal portions
3. Roll out a portion into a 200 mm diameter circle
4. Prick them all over using a fork and cut out into approximately small square pieces using a knife. You will get approximately 12 pieces
5. Repeat steps 3 and 4 to make 12 more pieces using another dough portion.
6. Arrange them on a greased baking tray and bake in a preheated oven at 180°c (360°f) for 25 to 30 minutes or till they turn crisp from both the sides, while turning them once after 12 minutes. Keep aside to cool slightly.
7. Store in an air-tight container and use as required.

Ingredients For The Ragi and Oat Crackers

1/2 cup ragi (nachni / red millet) flour
1/4 cup quick cooking rolled oats
1/2 cup whole wheat flour (gehun ka atta)
2 tsp olive oil
1/2 tsp green chili paste
1/2 tsp garlic (lehsun) paste salt to taste

To Be Mixed Into A Cucumber Dip
1/2 cup grated cucumber
1 cup hung low-fat curds (dahi) whisked
2 tbsp finely chopped mint leaves (phudina) leaves
2 tbsp finely chopped coriander (dhania)
1/4 tsp cumin seeds (jeera) powder
1/4 tsp garlic (lehsun) paste salt to taste Method For the ragi and oat crackers

Instructions
Combine all the ingredients in a deep bowl and knead into a stiff dough using enough water.
Divide the dough into 2 equal portions.
Roll out a portion into a 200 mm. diameter circle without using

any flour for rolling.
Prick them all over using a fork and cut into small squares
Arrange them on a greased baking tray and bake in a pre-heated oven at 180°c (360°f) for 25 to 30 minutes or till they turn crisp from both the sides, while turning them once after 12 minutes. Keep aside to cool slightly.

Veggies and Chicken Skillet

Ingredients:
All-purpose fl0ur, ¼ cup
Baby carrots, 2 oz
Cherry tomatoes, 1 cup
Finely chopped medium onion, 1 piece
Fresh sliced cremini mushroom, 7 oz
Ground pepper
Olive oil, 2 tbsp
Salt
Skinless and boneless chicken breasts, 14 oz
Vegetable or chicken stock, 1 cup
For garnish (optional): parsley, fresh

Instruction:
1. Pound chicken breasts until they are one inch thick. This will help the chicken cook evenly.
2. Put flour on a shallow plate. Add the salt pepper into the plate and then mix. Use this mixture to dredge the chicken breasts. Set aside.
3. Heat olive oil in a large skillet. Add the chicken breasts. Cook them until they start to look brown.
4. After this, set aside the chicken and put it in a plate.
5. In the same skillet pan, add the carrots, mushrooms, and onion. Sauté the ingredients for around 4-5 minutes. Add stock to cover up the chicken.
6. Let the stock come to a boil. Then, simmer with the lid on for 15-20 minutes
7. Lastly, add the cherry tomatoes and simmer. Wait until they have softened.
8. To garnish, just top the veggies and chicken skillet with the finely chopped fresh parsley.

Quinoa Tacos

Ingredients:
Quinoa
- White, tricolor, or red quinoa, 1 cup
- Vegetable broth or stock, 1 cup
- Water, ¾ cup

Seasonings
- Salsa with slightly chunky bits, ½ cup
- Nutritional yeast, 1 tbsp
- Ground cumin, 2 tsp
- Ground chili powder, 2 tsp
- Garlic powder, ½ tsp
- Sea salt, ½ tsp
- Black pepper, ½ tsp
- Avocado oil or olive oil, 1 tbsp

Instruction
1. Rinse quinoa beforehand. Heat a saucepan (medium-sized) over medium heat. When the pan is hot, put the quinoa then toast for around 4-5 minutes.
2. Pour water and vegetable broth. Bring it to a boil over medium-high heat. After boiling, reduce the heat to low and cook for 15-25 minutes with lid covered.
3. Fluff using a fork. Remove lid and remove from heat. Leave it to rest for 10 minutes.
4. Preheat your oven to 190 C (375 degrees F) at this point.
5. Add the cooked quinoa into a large mixing bowl. Put the salsa, cumin, nutritional yeast, chili powder, salt, pepper, garlic powder, and oil into the bowl with the cooked quinoa. Toss the ingredients
6. Line a parchment paper (or lightly greased) into a baking sheet. Spread the mixture in the sheet.
7. Bake the mixture for 20-35 minutes.

Baked Sweet Potato Fries

Ingredients
Large sweet potatoes, 2 pieces
Olive or coconut oil, 3 tbsp
Sea salt, ½ tsp
Ground black pepper, ½ tsp

Paprika, ¼ tsp

Instruction

1. Preheat oven to 450 degrees Fahrenheit.
2. Wash the sweet potatoes before using them. Pat them dry using napkins. Then, cut into half-inch slices, or how to think or thick you want your fries to be.
3. In a large mixing bowl, combine the sweet potatoes with oil.
4. Toss the ingredient in the bowl to coat all of the sweet potatoes.
5. Sprinkle salt, pepper, and paprika into the coated sweet potatoes.
6. Grease/ oil a baking sheet. Then, arrange the fries in a single layer with a little space between each.
7. Bake for around 18 to 25 minutes.

CONCLUSION

Fatty liver disease is an easily preventable and treatable condition and it doesn't even require expensive medication or treatment methods. Basically, the patient just needs to eat a healthy, balanced diet and indulge in exercise to lower body weight and improve liver health.

Avoid consuming highly-processed foods which are usually loaded with salt, sugar, and fats. Instead opt for whole foods, especially fruits and vegetables. Cutting down or completely abstaining from alcohol is also required.

As the saying goes, prevention is always better than the cure and the same applies to fatty liver. Eating healthy and exercising regularly should be a conscious choice. These ensure the protection of not only the liver, but the whole body as well.

Made in the USA
Coppell, TX
02 September 2021